Drawing the Line

Keyonna Murry

Drawing the Line

Copyright © 2020 by Keyonna M. Murry

The following work is a work of non-fiction. Information within this text is based on general knowledge acquired through education and experience. Any ideas and expressions are a product the author's personal thoughts and feelings.

ISBN-978-1-7351167-0-9

All rights reserved. No elements of this publication may be copied, scanned, or broadcasted on any platform, printed or digital, without written permission of the author.

www.drawingthelinewithlove.com

Cover Art by Taylor Jylha

About the Author

I am a righteous woman. I keep God first in my life. I allow my light to shine in spite of the darkness that encompasses the world. I allow people to see God in me, without offending or disregarding other's beliefs. I do not proclaim perfection nor stand before you stating that I have it all figured out. Even in my imperfections, I spread Love and promote growth. I am a queen, and nothing can make me feel inadequate. I can do all things through Christ who strengthens me. I am faithful, chosen, a role model, and leader. My beauty stems from the inside and emits through my eyes. I love you and I am praying for us as we learn to navigate the path to our purpose.

I dedicate this book to my grandma Marie. She taught me the beauty of writing and the power behind my words. Her letters will forever be in my heart and at the forefront of my thoughts.

Introduction

The emergency department is a controlled environment, no matter what happens around us. With sirens blaring, everyone may seem scattered, but we maintain control. We are expected to remain calm in the midst of chaos. With little to no training in handling this amount of pressure, somehow, I call commands in a code. I keep my composure, because the nurses that came to assist look to me for guidance.

In moments like this, I breathe deeply, and I take five seconds to process everything that is happening. I look around and wonder what everyone is thinking. My heart rate slows, I hear my breath with each inhalation and exhalation. *Do I pick up a pen or grab a syringe?* If I am the primary nurse, I pick up the pen. I do not want to find myself later having to piece together what occurred during the event. I need to record all the interventions carried out. If I am assisting, I pick up a syringe (or whatever the primary nurse needs). If no one is in control, I assign roles to ensure we maintain control. I never knew five seconds could feel so long.

Of course, it is not always a code situation in the emergency room. There are times of calm, but another nurse may have trouble. As an experienced nurse, I have an obligation to help and motivate others. Nursing is collaborative, and every member of the team plays their role. I examine my workload first, then help where I can. There certainly are times when I am the nurse in need of assistance.

The fast pace and high acuity can be overwhelming. Feeling like I was drowning, I looked for a lifeline, but no one could help. They were drowning as well. At my first nursing job, in the busiest emergency department in the city, I had an amazing preceptor. After introducing himself, his first words to me were, "Either you're going to sink, or you're going to swim." I often think back on those words. Initially, I was disappointed that he took this approach. With experience, I realized that he revealed the real world of emergency nursing to me.

    I had a lot to learn about nursing, starting with discovering how to use my voice. I needed to know how to prevent myself from sinking. I did not pretend to have the answers. If I was unfamiliar with a procedure or intervention, I vocalized it. I asked for help.

I chose a department with a climate that fostered an "everyone for themselves" mentality. As an emergency room nurse, I was expected to be highly skilled and self-efficient, skills I acquired as a military medical technician. But I wondered about those who did not share that experience.

I became an amazing nurse, developing a safe and effective approach to delivering patient care. This assisted me in navigating life. In learning to manage the pressures of dealing with high volume and acuity in the emergency department, I learned not to bring those problems home with me. I have applied that learning to calm any storms that rage in my life.

While my life is not perfect, I transition through life's seasons with ease, knowing I have a tool that sustains me. When I face issues, I feel more equipped to deal with them. I also have a clear mind and consciousness, because I put my heart into everything I do. Through "Seasons," I will share with you this tool.

Season 1

Self Love is the Best Love

Assessment *is the first step in the nursing process. In this stage of the process data gathering occurs. Nurses acquire the patient's perspective of their issues, subjective information. Then they complete a head-to-toe assessment that reveals visible issues, objective information. The patient's responses to questions during the gathering of subjective information and their reaction to commands given during the objective information gathering provides ques to the nurse of which disease process is taking place. Assessment is a pathway for nurses to recognize any issues that require immediate attention and obtain a complete understanding of the nature of the reason behind a patient's visit. An assessment establishes the framework and foundation for the rest of the visit*

When you look in the mirror what do you see? What is your perception of yourself? What do you dislike about yourself? What do you love about yourself? What is visible to others when they look at you? These are questions that can be used to assess yourself. Assessment is a systemic method to collect physiological and psychological information and use it the evaluate issues discovered. Love is a concept that is grown into. In order to grow and progress in love, assessment has to take place.

Love is patient, Love is kind, Love is forgiving, Love is not boastful, Love is not proud. In this journey, Love is what sustains and fulfills us. Love is defined as an intense feeling of deep affection. Love is unconditional, meaning that no matter what the circumstance it won't disappear. Acquiring true Love is something that most people struggle with but that does not mean that it is not attainable. There is also more to Love than feeling affection. It is an emotion that drives us in the way that we interact with people, live our lives, and make decisions.

Love is a feeling that needs to be emitted into the world in action. The understanding of Love establishes the foundation. Correlating Love to life is what helps us navigate the path and encounters along the way to our destiny. Love possesses power that is often under utilized. On this journey there will be storms that discourage, derail, hurt, and disappoint us. Acknowledgement of these trials activates Love's full power. In these times, Love will give us comfort and strength to propel forward. Love will console us and allow thoughts of peace to surround the chaos. We are not alone in our walk.

People are designed to live in union. Often times, this is analyzed as meaning with another person. The reality is that people are designed to live in union with Love. It is important to confess that this journey, known as life, cannot be conquered alone. Admitting that life is difficult and we need help makes room in our lives for Love. Love will help us make it through the storm. There has to be a desire to know Love in order to grow in Love. After discovering what Love is, allow it to flow into action. Be patient. Be kind. Be forgiving. Do not be boastful. Do not walk in pride. When we look in the mirror, there should be a reflection of Love.

Love is an easy concept, but we complicate it by searching for it in other and expecting others to provide it for us. We have control over what we pour our love into and the way we use it, start with ourselves. Nurses are taught to complete a head-to-toe assessment to assess patients' functionality and identify any abnormalities. This method of assessment can be used be a common person to identify areas among themselves where love is needed.

Love needs to be fostered from the inside and embracement of surface level flaws will occur. Look into your eyes, they are the window to our souls. Do the thoughts and emotions that reside there align with Love? The light of the body is in the eyes, if light is present in the eyes, the whole body is full of light. Love provides clarity in dark times. If we look into our eyes and discover darkness allow Love to radiate light. Replace those thoughts with truth, what is noble, whatever is pure, whatever is lovely, whatever is admirable, and things that are excellent and praiseworthy. We may not be where we want to be in life, but we have made it to this point. There are small accomplishments that are overlooked at times because of their size. Learn to embrace the smaller things achieved in life and the appreciation for greater things will increase, but more importantly there will be a new level of satisfaction within our souls and light that overcasts the darkness.

The head-to-toes assessment is sequential, now assess our heart. Many cultures symbolize Love with a heart. The synonymous use of Love and heart reminds us that this is where our morals and values lie. Our heart is what propels us into action based on our ideal of love. On a deeper level of understanding, Love differentiates right from wrong. The heart and soul have a complicated relationship. Thoughts and emotions stem from the mind. The heart is built upon

Love. When darkness encompasses the soul, it is difficult for the heart to be on the same accord. The heart tells us that feelings of darkness are not welcome. The heart attempts to show the mind how to access the light, but sometimes we block our own light. Is your heart and mind of the same accord? If not remind yourself of the principles that Love has instilled in your heart. If it does not feel right, follow your intuition to work toward fixing the issue.

Nurses will ask patients to extend their arms to assess their strength with lifting and ability to maintain this position against gravity. The importance of discovering Love within ourselves and understanding the function of it is to adequately equip us to extend it to others. If the dark places in our soul remain unaddressed it will reflect in the way we care for others. The way that we understand Love within ourselves and provide it for ourselves is the way we project it unto others. Loving ourselves and understanding what Love is strengthens us to reach out and touch others. The more we grow in Love, the more we will understand that satisfaction with life does not arise from what we can do for ourselves, but what we are capable of doing for others. Gravity is a natural phenomenon that brings things toward one another.

The union with Love should be able to withstand the forces of gravity. We encounter multitudes of people on a daily basis. Some will have similar values and beliefs and others may have opposing beliefs. The understanding of how Love resonates within us should grow but not change. our union with Love is unique. It belongs to you and you only. Defend your union with Love, but also respect others union. We are capable of living and working together for the greater good with opposing or different beliefs. Learn to coexist.

The last thing assessed in a head-to-toe assessment is the feet. We use our feet to move. Walking with Love is exercising the power Love possesses. Once we have a clear understanding of what love is, apply it to ourselves, and develop a desire to extend it to others we allow our actions to reflect Love. Love is perfect, but we are not. Along the way mistakes will be made, do not allow fear to bind you from taking steps forward in your journey. The bigger picture may not be clear in the moment but allow Love to lead the way. When we feel an urge to move, will us take those steps? Love will not fail us.

Explore the depths of Love until you have a clear understanding. Everyone has a purpose on earth. Some discover their purpose sooner than others. An assessment of your heart and soul will reveal your purpose. It is not an easy task and transformation will not take place overnight. If a clear purpose does not present itself upon your assessment, understand that everyone's purpose is to love. The nursing process is an organized process that requires specific thought and each step builds on information from the prior step.

Assessment is the first step in the process. We collect information that can be useful in leading to the next step of the process. If our purpose is to Love, we have to accept that we will have to carry this out even in our imperfections. We all have flaws, acknowledging your flaws makes application of

Love less difficult. All of the answers will not be provided when walking in Love. We do not have control over our journey and the roads we are led down and decide to take. It is okay to not have control. The admission of no control is having total control in situations. Choose peace over control. Displacement of emotions and thoughts hold us captive, therefore be considerate of your thoughts and what you allow to resonate in your soul.

    The assessment reveals our strengths and weaknesses. It exposes things that we may not have been aware of prior to completing a head-to-toe assessment. Our perspective of what is going on is a guide to narrow the possibilities. It is not until a full assessment is complete that we obtain the objective information needed to combine with the subjective that will lead us to diagnosing a problem. How often are you assessing yourself? People come to the hospital when they are not well. We should not wait until we are in distress to assess ourselves. An assessment can take place as often as we think about it but it is imperative when we feel lost or off track that we take the time to do a head-to-toe.

Love has no limits and will not always be reciprocated. After assessing the psychological elements of who you are, identify physical limitations. Choosing peace over chaos, protects you from experiencing darkness from things that are out of your control. Physical limitations place limits on what you can accomplish physically and makes the psychological transformation more difficult. Instead of focusing on what cannot be accomplished because of limitations, place emphasis on what can be done with your limitations.

Assessments are the foundation of the nursing process. Each step in the process is built on the information and data collected in the assessment. The same sequence an assessment is carried out in nursing can be used in life. Collect subjective information, the patients'/ your perception of the problem. Then gather objective data. The difference in applying this tool to life is that a head-to-toe assessment is used to collect physiological and psychological information about yourself, as opposed to it only being used in the objective gathering information in nursing. Your assessment will reveal areas of yourself that can potentially cause deep seeded issues if they go unaddressed, bind you, prevent you from progressing in life and relationships. Love is capable of healing all wounds, but there has to a clear understanding of it and the desire to act within it. Understanding love is a process that takes time and requires nurturing roots to promote growth. Once fulfilled with Love in ourselves, a desire to extend it to others should develop in spite of our differences we should be able to stand on Love and share it freely. It is not our responsibility to make others see Love in the same light as us, but we should emit our light in a way that prompts others to find the light in themselves.

Nurses are trained in completing head-to-toe assessments on others that are under their care. Do not attempt to complete a head-to-toe assessment on others, lead them to trained professionals. It is okay to recommend therapy to people in your life that you are concerned about. Full comprehension of Love is not easy; therefore, some will need help coming to terms with what Love is and its power. Be a light in the same manner you should be for yourself when you experience dark thoughts and emotions. You cannot fix or change others, Love can. Do not be selfish with your Love. Share Love with the world, even those that have hurt you. There is liberation in the proper use of Love.

Journal Entry

I have walked past the mirror countless times. Yesterday was the first time I truly looked in the mirror and saw who I had become. The last time I evaluated myself I was more confident in my appearance. I recall seeing a girl who had it all figured out. Accomplished, wise beyond her year of age, beautiful, and ready to take on the world. Yesterday, I still saw those characteristics, but some traits were unfamiliar. Along the journey to my purpose, there was a shift in my character. I no longer felt impactful. I noticed that I had become more self-conscious and questioned my true capabilities. I'm slowly losing site of the path I have chosen, but still holding on to my morals and values.

Season 2

Hope is More Powerful than Fear

Diagnosis *is the identification of the problem. Nurses make an educated judgement using the data collected in the assessment to ascertain potential or actual problems. A diagnosis goes beyond recognizing a problem, it reveals risks for developing complications and it determines readiness for health improvement. A diagnosis provides clarity on the appropriate pathway to choose that is capable of addressing identified issues. There are specific pathways associated with diseases that are supported by evidence that will guide healthcare providers through delivering appropriate interventions and improving health outcomes. There can be multiple diagnosis based upon the information gathered during the assessment. Nurses are provided a list of diagnosis* *that encompass Maslow's Hierarchy of Needs, prioritization of basic fundamental needs innate for all.* Maslow suggests that basic physiologic needs must be met before higher needs can be achieved. Physiological and safety establish the basis for nursing interventions and are the foundation for physical and emotional health. A diagnosis assists in distinguishing what patients are up against.

Fear arises in the face of uncertainty and the unknown. Fear is an emotion that hinders us from living in our purpose. Action does not have to be placed behind fear, redirect that action into love. The only thing stronger than fear is hope. Hope will cast out any fear that manifests in your life. Choose hope over fear. Do not allow fear to cast doubt in your mind, you can do whatever you set your mind to but make sure that you do it in love. Hope is derived from knowing or having an idea of what the problem is. Hope is more powerful than fear, because hope is a product of love and unbinds us from anything keeping us bound.

After completing the head-to-toe assessment where did the problems lay? When you explored your soul did you have distorted thoughts, were you confused about your emotions? What is the foundation of your morals and values? Do you have a desire to help others? Do you listen to your intuition when it is telling you to move?

You may not be educated in nursing diagnoses, but you have experience that can be a basis for your diagnoses. Signs and symptoms of troubles you may have experienced in the past or seen others struggle with may present themselves and hopefully you will be able to recognize them.

The beauty of diagnoses is that you do not have to get it correct the first time. Taking the initiative to assess yourself and place a label on a potential issue or issue you are experiencing leads to self-improvement. You love yourself enough to acknowledge the voice telling you that something is not right, and you are driven to heal those wounds causing pain and destruction in your life. You may discover things about yourself that you are not ready to face, those are barriers.

    Beyond diagnosing concerns within, barriers also need to be identified and diagnosed. Barriers prevent us from moving forward along our destined path. They limit our abilities and potential. Placing barriers in a category takes away their power. We recognize that they are barriers and we will find a way to overcome them or ways if we are not successful in our first attempt. There will be many obstacles along the journey living in your purpose. Those obstacles are not meant break or destroy us, there is something to be learned in overcoming obstacles and barriers.

Love teaches us dependency, which is why establishing a higher understanding of Love is imperative. When we reach roadblocks, we have to diagnose them. Coming to terms with barriers we may have created, is one of the most difficult tasks in the diagnosis phase. We do not like being wrong or admitting that we are the one's stopping ourselves from our destiny. Barriers are inevitable, but do not equate to an end. After overcoming the barriers we encounter, we can continue on our journey and deal with the issues that lay ahead.

The thoughts that we allow to consume our minds that do not align with our heart are a problem. Hopelessness, fear, depression, unsatisfaction, are problems that we face in the world. We are subject to human desires and emotions, but we have power over which ones we allow to occupy our minds and hearts. We all have problems that we are battling on a daily basis. Do not feel like you are alone in the fight. We are discovering good and bad things about ourselves through assessment. The same manner that we accept the good we see within, is the same manner that needs to be applied to transform the bad. Isolation is a place of destruction; it is not a place for us but rather a place for our problems.

Diagnoses isolate our problems and expose them for what they are. Once you acquire a higher understanding of love and allow it to flow into action it will never leave you. It will help you work through issues you are having with yourself or those around you. It's okay to depend on love and explore the depths of your soul. Identifying things that are holding you back will become more visible. At times you will come to the discovery that the issue may not be you, it may be people you allow in your space. Isolation of issues makes it clear where the root of the problem stems.

      Problems will keep you content where you are. There is a difference in being satisfied and being content. Growth in love leads to satisfaction. Being content leads to complacency and presents fear an invitation to enter our minds. Fear keeps you in bondage. Diagnosing problems allow us to see the problem and provides pathways to resolving them. Allow the power of hope to intercede on your part. Hope will provide pathways like diagnoses provide guidance for nurses.

If a diagnosis for which you are experiencing does not exist already, create one. There are guidelines for diagnosing in nursing but there are none for diagnosing life issues. We are in control of our souls and hearts. What we allow to enter does not equate allowing it to occupy. Recognizing the problem in this step of the process. It is important that identification is made because that will guide the route to resolving the issue. This process can be started as many times necessary to fix the discovered issues. In this stage of the process it is okay to admit you do not have all the answers. It is the determination to discover what went wrong and the driving force behind learning from your mistakes. There is freedom and identifying our problems there is freedom in exploring pathways for a better life for satisfaction with our transformation.

Journal Entry

I could not have dreamed the life that I am currently living. My reality surpassed my goals. I remained strong in my faith and allowed it to guide me through life. Yet, it still does not feel like I've done enough. I was watching a television show that discussed **imposter syndrome,** *a collection of feelings of inadequacy that persist despite evident success.* My fear of failing and not meeting the expectations others placed on me allowed doubt to enter my mind. I push myself too hard in every aspect of my life because

I've convinced myself that failure is not an option. I've placed other's expectations of me ahead of my own. Instead of embracing the support I've received, I spend the majority of my time working to prove those that don't believe in me wrong.

Season 3

Place of Preparation

Planning *is the phase where a plan of action is developed to work through the identified problems. Pathways for issues are designed and prioritized based on the highest risk for danger. Clear measurable goals are established that align with beneficial outcomes. The goals range from short-term to long-term goals. These goals are derived from specific pathways associated with identified problems and built around the patient's capabilities. The goals are specific, measurable, attainable, result producing, and timely oriented.*

Planning is a highly effective method that aids in getting through the process of healing. The place of preparation is where structure is established for interventions that we carry out to propel through our journey. Planning reveals available resources, organizes interventions, and provides direction on the destination we are attempting to reach. It also will help us achieve our goals and clearly present our options if our problem is not resolved with our first intervention. It will motivate us through the process because we have also identified our options.

The place of preparation is a very difficult place to be in. It requires patience and understanding of the transformation in our lives without knowing the final product. We have to acknowledge and recognize that the place of preparation is not meant to destroy us, but to restructure us. We are reclaiming our peace and satisfaction with where we are in life. We are planning to leave the place of preparation better than how we entered it. We establish a plan of action based on our resources and capabilities. The place of preparation is where we have to remind ourselves of the Love, we instilled in ourselves. Then we must remind ourselves of the things Love possesses to drive our plan of action. How will we confront our problems? What actions do we need to include in our plan to progress in our journey? How will our actions benefit our mental health and the world?

In the place of preparation, we need to discover an increased hunger to live in our purpose. The goals designed during the planning phase should be meaningful, attainable, and realistic. Unlike in nursing practice there does not have to be time limits placed on when these goals are achieved. The journey we are on is about growth. We produce growth by continually working on the person we are in the world ensuring our actions align with Love. We do not have all the answers, or everything figured out. The intention of resolving an issue we see within ourselves leads to a better life.

Address issues that place you at risk for the greatest harm to yourself or others first. There is a possibility that by addressing these issues, a snowball effect can occur and resolve issues associated with the problem. Trust the process. It is important in these stages that we create pathways associated with problems we found in ourselves that are tailored to us. We have resources that have named problems similar to what we are experiencing, but we have to personalize those pathways to address what we are experiencing. The reality is what helped others resolve their issues, may not be the solution to our problem. We need to also consider the affect our problems have on others and include resolution in our plans.

    Goals address self-improvement but are also a platform for atonement. At times, the pain we imposed on others can be a problem that is weighing us down or impeding our progress. Love teaches us forgiveness. Once we have forgiven ourselves for our past actions and our role in hurting others, it can be an action in our plan to restoration and healing. We are more likely to work toward goals that are meaningful to us. Establishing a meaningful goal provides incentive to follow through with plans to acquire it. When we set unrealistic goals for ourselves, we are setting ourselves up for destruction. There is action that takes place in the next phase of the nursing process, if our goals are unrealistic, that energy goes into empty space that leaves residuals of disappointment. Goals should be specific in nature, so that what we are willing to do to resolve this problem is visible and clear in our plan.

Time- oriented goals are beneficial pertaining to work and things of the world. There is no time limit that can be placed on our healing. It is nice to have short-term and long-term goals associated with actions we are working toward healing, but healing is a product of growth. The more we grow in Love, the more we will come to the realization that pain is a part of the process. There is a purpose for your pain, the place of preparation reveals what you have made room for in your life. It is where we make a decision to improve our lives. The place of preparation is where we break chains that have been holding us back from living in our purpose. We embrace pain in this phase because we know it will push us into our purpose.

A plan illustrates what can be done to free us from bondage. We create this plan based on our resources and abilities. All things learned and understood about Love is what should be the foundation of our plans. Our goals should be established around our growth and understanding of Love. As simple as this may sound, Love is capable of solving all our problems. The power in Love is provided for those that seek it. Planning is the pathway to success.

We all have a version of success that only we can achieve. We must set ourselves up for success through planning. In order to accomplish this during the planning phase, we have to define success. The way we define success in our lives pertaining to problems we are confronting are objectives. When battling depression, we should have an object that aligns with happiness and light that emphasizes the need to decrease isolation. Isolating ourselves during hard times can lead to darkness. We must formulate a plan that allows the light within us to shine. Love is the light that emits rays that illuminate the darkness. Anger, revenge, depression, and hate are products of darkness. In our planning we have to consider all things dimming our light and manifest a pathway that will recharge our light.

Planning allows us to see the light within us. It reminds us of all the things we learned in Love that are more powerful than what darkness can bring. Love is patient; therefore, during the planning phase formulate a plan that will lead you to be more patient with whatever you are battling or waiting for. Establish a pathway to step aside from what is dimming your light. Plan to walk in love. Plan to be the light, that others cannot see in themselves. Map out ways to share your light with the world but be careful not to become of the world. We have to remain faithful and true to who we are in Love.

It is important to grasp the idea that there is no action required in this phase of the process. The place of preparation is where we mentally prepare to activate our power in healing our wounds. Before placing action behind our plans, we have to mentally prepare ourselves for the outcomes. The reality is that our plans may not lead to resolution or healing. The preparation in this phase is beyond encouraging ourselves to move but also sustaining ourselves in the face of failure and disappointment. It is not about how many times we fall down; it is about how we get up and carry on. Love will sustain us in the transition from the place of preparation into the implementation phase.

Love is a source of power. Everyone may not have the same belief as us, but Love is universal. In order to advance through the preparation phase of the process we have to be on the same wavelength as our source of power. Our source of power will teach us how to adequately plan for our purpose and equip us with all that we need. If we discover our purpose in the place of preparation some of us may not feel qualified. This feeling leads to further dependence on Love. We want to be vulnerable with our source of power because we channel power within ourselves from Love. We must align ourselves with Love because it will bare us for who we are and not who we pretend to be. We have to reclaim our power in the place of preparation because we will need it to move into action.

Planning and proper preparation will allow you to feel when it is time to put your plans into action. It is imperative that you have a desire to change and move forward in the healing process. The implementation phase cannot be forced. We have to have a will to grow in Love. Plan like you know when the time to move is coming, so that when it arises within us, we are ready. The transformation happens within you so that Love can be projected through you.

Journal Entry

I will embrace every accomplishment, no matter the size. I will change the way I perceive failure. There is something to be learned in making mistakes. An error is an opportunity for improvement and growth. I will take other's expectations of me as a compliment and set my own. When doubt begins to enter my mind, I will reflect on my accomplishments. I will remind myself that if I made it through previous difficult situations, I can make it through the one I am facing. I will replace fear with hope and allow Love to intercede on my behalf. I will always make room for more and no longer be bound to marginalization. I will listen to my soul when it tells me, slow down.

Season 4

The Healing Garden

Implementation *is the phase of the process when plans are put into action. The plans created in the planning phase are launched in attempt to achieve desired outcomes. During this phase an assessment of the interventions take place that help transition to other developed interventions if the one in use does not appear to be effective. Implementation of planned interventions requires monitoring for changes and improvements. Achieving goals can occur in hours, days, weeks, months, even years depending on continuity of care. This is the action phase.*

Everything that we formulated during the planning phase is imperative to our healing. Take note of the intentional use of healing as opposed to fixing. Our goals are aimed toward healing wounds and addressing issues that we have within ourselves. It is important to remember that we are aiming for a better life and sometimes that requires us to live with disabilities and predisposed issues. Transformation begins in the mind.

The first three steps of the nursing process are tools that help transform the mind. First, we completed a subjective and objective assessment of who we are. Second, we diagnosed issues that we found during our assessment. Lastly, we began planning the pathway to resolve our issues within. These steps mentally prepare us for the steps we will take to improve who we are. In the process we also made a decision, either we will walk in light or remain bound to the wars of our world. Love radiates light.

Radiation of our light depends on our belief in Love's power. Love's purpose is to be our power, confidence and freedom. When we choose Love, we choose to walk in a life that is radiant. There will be seasons that block the light from fully radiating, but the light never leaves. In these seasons do not try to force action, there is nothing that can be done to prevent the season from occurring or shorten it. Seasons pass and Love remains present and faithful. In those seasons of disappointment, pain, and suffering be present and allow it to produce growth. In order for plants to grow they need light, water, and attention.

The healing garden is a mental place composed of Love. I feel closest to my source of power when I am near water. It is the most powerful element on earth. Bodies of water are designed to flow with the wind. On the surface water can appear calm, but an aquatic kingdom exists in the depths of it. Water has the ability to freeze into a solid element, produces growth in plantation, and flushes out impurities in the human body. It can also be destructive during storms and hurricanes. When water is visible, I feel a transference of power. It reminds me that I possess control over my decisions and power to be a light when darkness casts my thoughts.

Love is a spring of water and provides moisture to the dry areas in our lives. Even when we take a sip of water, that is sufficient to sustain us on our journey. The amount of water a plant needs varies based on the type. Love produces small, moderate, and life changing plants in our lives. The garden symbolizes the manifestation of harvest that stems from the roots we planted with Love. Anger, revenge, bitterness, and hatred will cause decomposition in your garden when action is placed behind them instead of replacement.

It is natural to experience feelings of anger and pain. It is not natural to be encompassed by darkness. The longer we allow darkness to block our light the tighter the chains become in bondage. Anger, fear, and hatred bind us. You have to choose freedom and the path requires Love. It takes more energy to carry out these negative emotions because they have power over us and consume our minds. Love in the face of pain is a more difficult action to carry out but there is a reward that allows our souls to rest. It is natural to want to hurt others when we have been hurt, but we have to show them our light.

The healing garden needs light to prosper. Light is a source of energy that promotes growth in plants. Our mind is a foundation for growth. We have control over what we believe and disregard. Sometimes it takes others to push us into our purpose. There may be someone that supports and believes in your abilities more than you at the moment. There may also be someone that doesn't believe you are capable of achieving your goals. Both scenarios can be the driving force behind propelling you forward. Never allow either case to be the reason behind action. Do it for yourself or do it for Love. No one can walk in your purpose but you. They may be motivation, but the walk is yours. We are in constant battle with ourselves about what we are being called to do or our purpose.

Implementing the plans, we created to heal our wounds may not take effect overnight. This is why during the planning phase we need to mentally prepare ourselves for results that may not be favorable. We do not stop at the inability of our plan to heal us. We have to implement the next plan. Walking with Love guides us through growth and is everything we need. When we are weak, Love is strong. We are breaking chains one link at a time. The ability to move forward with pain, anger, and sorrow pulling at our feet is strength. One step at a time. Acknowledge and celebrate the small victories because this will increase your strength. What we lack in strength, Love will compensate. The stronger we get, the easier it will be to walk in our light.

Implementing the plans is progression in our journey. We cannot allow fear to hinder us from propelling forward. Implementing things of Love will lead to higher regard for others. We are not fulfilled by the things we do for ourselves, but our ability to do for others. In order to give Love, we have to know Love within. Once we implement plans that develop Love within us, it will begin to show in our actions. The way we treat people is a reflection of our sense of Love within and our understanding of its power.

The challenge of doing for others is reciprocity. The reality is that while we may be beacons of light, others may not be in the same place in their walk. Never expect reciprocity. Carry out Love with the expectation of dispersing it and not always receiving it. We never know the impact of loving someone who does not know Love or hasn't been shown genuine Love. The reward is an improved version of who we see in the mirror. We seek validation from others, but the only validation we need is from Love. "I love me enough to strive to be better than I was yesterday." One day at a time.

We almost must center our focus on our core. Throughout this process we have been preparing our minds and hearts to act in a capacity that improves who we are. We have to focus on ourselves. During implementation it is very easy to look at others' success and failures and began to compare them to our plans. The key is to remember that we are walking in a lane designed for ourselves. No one can occupy the path we are destined for. The same applies to those around us. Their journey will not look exactly like ours. We cannot fall into the trap of comparison, this will hinder our walk. It will decrease our confidence and may slow us down in implementing the plans we have designed to succeed. People will have similar experiences that will be relatable, but they cannot be the foundation for our implementation.

The foundation of our implementation is Love. We acknowledge this and keep this at the forefront of our minds when carrying out action. First, we attained a higher understanding of Love. Second, we explored our minds and hearts to reveal any deficits and discrepancies, so that we could apply Love to ourselves. Third, we formulated a plan on how to heal and move forward in our journey. Now, we are walking in Love.

It is important to be present in our actions. We have to take note on the impact walking in Love has on not only ourselves, but those around us. Springing into action and allowing the fruits of Love to come to fruition has an effect on everyone. There should be a shift in your heart and mind. All things will not be perfect, but it should feel easier.

Journal Entry

Writing plans to improve who I am provided me visibility of what I was facing. I see the problem. Now, I am ready to begin the healing process. I am not capable of carrying out all of my plans in this moment, but I am preparing myself for when the time comes. I revised my resume and applauded myself for my accomplishments. I also read old journal entries and realized how far I've come from the girl I used to be. I see a blossoming rose in uncommon circumstances. I set goals five years ago and accomplished them *all. Today, I wrote new ones. I still fear failing, but when I encounter it I plan on embracing it with the intent of learning.*

Season 5

Self-Reflection

Evaluation *is the final step of the nursing process. After applying all the principles in the nursing process, this step determines if interventions were effective and if there was improvement in the patient's condition. An assessment if goals were met occurs. All that is known about the patient, their condition, and the nurses' previous experience is calculated to determine the effectiveness of care.*

Do you understand what Love is? Is Love the foundation you are building on? Are you content with what you see in the mirror? Have you acknowledged all of your problems? Do roadblocks exist that prevent you from moving forward? Are your plans adequate for your diagnoses? Is your healing process healthy? Did you produce fruits of Love? Do others see Love in you?

This is the stage of exploration. Some of our plans may have not worked out during the process. This stage is where we figure out what we did incorrect in the process. We also formulate methods to improve what did not work. We reflect on our understanding of Love and if the application of it in life is sufficient to sustain us upon our journey. Along the journey to restoration and happiness we may have developed new habits or experienced events that led to the development of unwanted feelings. The most important aspect of this stage is acknowledging that this journey is an ongoing learning process. Our interventions may be effective in this season of our lives, but may not work along the road. We take this time to grow in our position. There is always room for improvement. We have to assess what we have made room for in our lives.

Do not be afraid to let things go that hinder your growth. Eliminating those people and things will make room for what you have learned along the way to manifest. Whether we were successful or not., we commend ourselves for attempting. An attempt is a stride toward improvement.

Reflection is how we acknowledge our effort to emit Love. We start with evaluating how we feel about ourselves. If we are not content with how we treat ourselves or our values, we have to revisit what we learned about Love and plan a different approach at applying it to ourselves. We also must acknowledge the things we may have missed or suppressed. In life we can develop the tendency to normalize behaviors or things that cause anger, frustration, pain, or heartache. It is important to evaluate the diagnosis we placed upon ourselves. As we work through resolving issues, we often times will discover that based on the additional information and our responses to interventions, that we may have incorrectly diagnosed ourselves.

If our diagnoses were incorrect, that could explain why some of our interventions were not effective. After evaluating how we display Love internally, the diagnoses we have given ourselves, and the interventions toward healing we use that same process to assess how we have shown Love to others. Using the nursing process to guide us through life not only improves the quality of our lives, but it also impacts those around us.

We have to ensure that we have forgiven those who caused us physical or emotional harm. In the process we may have felt as though this was not necessary considering the amount of damage imposed on us. We may have felt like those people are beyond the point of reconciliation. Forgiveness is not for those who harmed us, it is for ourselves. It takes more energy to harbor hate than it does to radiate Love. We have to be cognoscente of the way we allow others to treat us. We have transformed our minds and stand on Love, therefore we should not allow others to mistreat us because of their position or relationship with us. The people around us need to treat us the same way we treat them. We must be a walking display of Love, in hopes that it will prompt others to explore themselves and strive toward doing the same.

    The evaluation phase is not encompassed around what was done wrong. We also evaluate the things that went well during the process. Life has a way of repeating lessons or experiences. This phase of the process is where we gather tools that we will equip ourselves with if we encounter similar situations. If we begin to notice drifts in our peace and happiness, we will use the tools that brought us to equilibrium to shift back in balance. If we notice toxic traits and behaviors from others, we have the courage to use our voice and we can rest confident in the fact that we are speaking from Love. The evaluation phase is where we develop a plan to maintain balance.

We develop a strategy that transitions us into what comes next. An evaluation of our morals and beliefs occur. Love should lead us to something greater than ourselves. We reflect on who we have become and if we are content with the way we handle situations in our lives. We evaluate peace, freedom, hope, and righteousness because these are the products of Love. Through walking in Love, we develop the ability to place fruits of Love on a scale. This is where we define if we are comfortable with our levels of Love. We assess if we possess all four or if we are deficient. If we find ourselves happy with the scale, we evaluate how to maintain and progress. If we are dissatisfied with where the scale aligns, we evaluate how we ended up there and what we are going to do to progress.

    A progression map is created in the evaluation phase. Reflecting on the process we progress forward in the cycle of the nursing process. Reflection occurs throughout the entire nursing process but during the evaluation phase it is done a deeper level. In this stage we are reclaiming our power over ourselves. We take this moment to reflect on the entire process and how far we have come, then we strategize to continue on our journey. We are in control of our decisions and this is where we reflect on our transformation.

Righteousness is hard to maintain in the world where there is so much destruction going on around us. It is easy to feel despair when the world appears to be crumbling in the enemies' favor. Love teaches us that justice will prevail. We take in consideration the environment we are in, the people in our lives, our position, social status, race, and religion but we do not allow these things to determine who we are. We have to stand firm on Love and allow others to see it within us. We must also establish our source of power so that when the road we choose is leading to despair that we are given assurance that the season will pass. We cannot become what the world wants us to be. We have to be who we are in spite of what anyone says. Even when no one applauds our good deeds and progression, we still have to walk in Love. We have to look ourselves in the mirror and be okay with what we have dispersed into the universe. If we are not able to look at ourselves in the mirror, we will not be at peace.

Journal Entry

Love possesses the power to sustain me through difficult times. It is the light that emits in the midst of darkness. When I find myself sinking, Love is the raft that keeps me afloat. It is what I see when I look in the mirror and what others see when they look at me. I may not be where I want to be, but I am far from what I used to be. I cannot make everyone happy. I realize it is okay to put myself first at times. I've compiled methods that displace fear of failing. I say I accept that I do not have all the answers, but I am willing to search for them. I'm appreciative of high expectations. It is a reflection of the hard work and dedication I put into my work. Who would have thought a troubled young girl would blossom into a beautiful rose in her older years.

Walk with Love

Grasping the true meaning of Love and developing a relationship with Love is the easiest path to perfect peace. Life will not be perfect but when we find ourselves in a whirlwind, we can rest knowing that Love will sustain us. Perfect peace is the alleviation of responsibility for things beyond our control. We learn to accept who we are and equip ourselves for the path destined for us. We do not hold ourselves accountable for others' actions. We know that they are granted the same choices we have in life and we cannot lead them down the same path that we are on.

Perfect peace presents through Love because we no longer compare our progress to others. We are in union with Love and will encounter others with a similar relationship along the way. We are not alone in our walk. Establishing a relationship with Love ensures that when all things and people fail us, it will still be present. When we feel too weak to continue through obstacle, Love will be our strength. Walking in Love leads to liberation.

      Love possesses the power to break chains. It protects us from the world, but most importantly ourselves. Sadly, we can be our biggest enemy. We place limitations on ourselves and doubt our capabilities but growing in Love can resolve that. As we foster growth and develop a higher understanding of Love, we restore our faith in ourselves. It is easy to get complacent in our journey. We know how easy it is to be of the world, but we walk in truth and spirit. In spite of what others say about us or our abilities, we are ourselves because we know Love. A higher understanding of

Love will reveal who you truly are. The relationship with Love releases us from bondage that tradition and the world has placed on us. We do not live according to society, but what we Love. Hope arises from knowing that there is more to come.

Even when we are not able to see the bigger picture, Love is interceding on our part. The outcome may not be clear, but we trust the process. We may go through seasons of disappointment, pain, and sadness, but with Love we know that it will pass. Hope is more powerful than fear. Walking with Love produces the confident expectation that we are capable of succeeding. We carry out acts with thoughts of succeeding as opposed to failure. Even if we find ourselves unsuccessful, we are able to process it as a learning moment with the tools that we acquired from utilizing the nursing process.

The nursing process is a tool that was developed to assist nurses in managing and delivering patient care, but it possesses far more capabilities. The nursing process can guide, those who are willing to apply it to life, through the journey of restoration. It will not be a perfect walk, but it will be an impactful one. Building on Love allows products of Love to manifest. We walk in our purpose while allowing Love to radiate into the world. It is easier said than done, but all of us are capable of using this tool. Let's begin at **Step one.**

When you look in the mirror what do you see? What is your perception of yourself? What do you dislike about yourself? What do you love about yourself? What is visible to others when they look at you?

What is the problem? What is preventing you from discovering your purpose and living in it?

_____

_____

_____

_____

_____

_____

_____

_____

_____

_____

_After completing the head-to-toe assessment where did the problems lay? When you explored your soul did you have distorted thoughts, were you confused about your emotions? What is the foundation of your morals and values? Do you have a desire to help others? Do you listen to your intuition when it is telling you to move?

_____

_____

_____

_____

_____

_____

_____

_____

How will you confront your problems? What actions do you need to include in your plan to progress in your journey? How will your actions benefit your mental health and the world?

_____

_____

_____

_____

_____

_____

_____

_____

_____

_____

_____

What steps will you take to mentally prepare yourself for the steps you will take to improve who you are?

Do you understand what Love is? Is Love the foundation you are building on? Are you content with what you see in the mirror? Have you acknowledged all of your problems? Do roadblocks exist that prevent you from moving forward? Are your plans adequate for your diagnoses? Is your healing process healthy? Did you produce fruits of Love? Do others see Love in you?

Love never fails. But where there are prophecies, they will cease; where there are tongues, they will be stilled; where there is knowledge, it will pass away.

Thank You

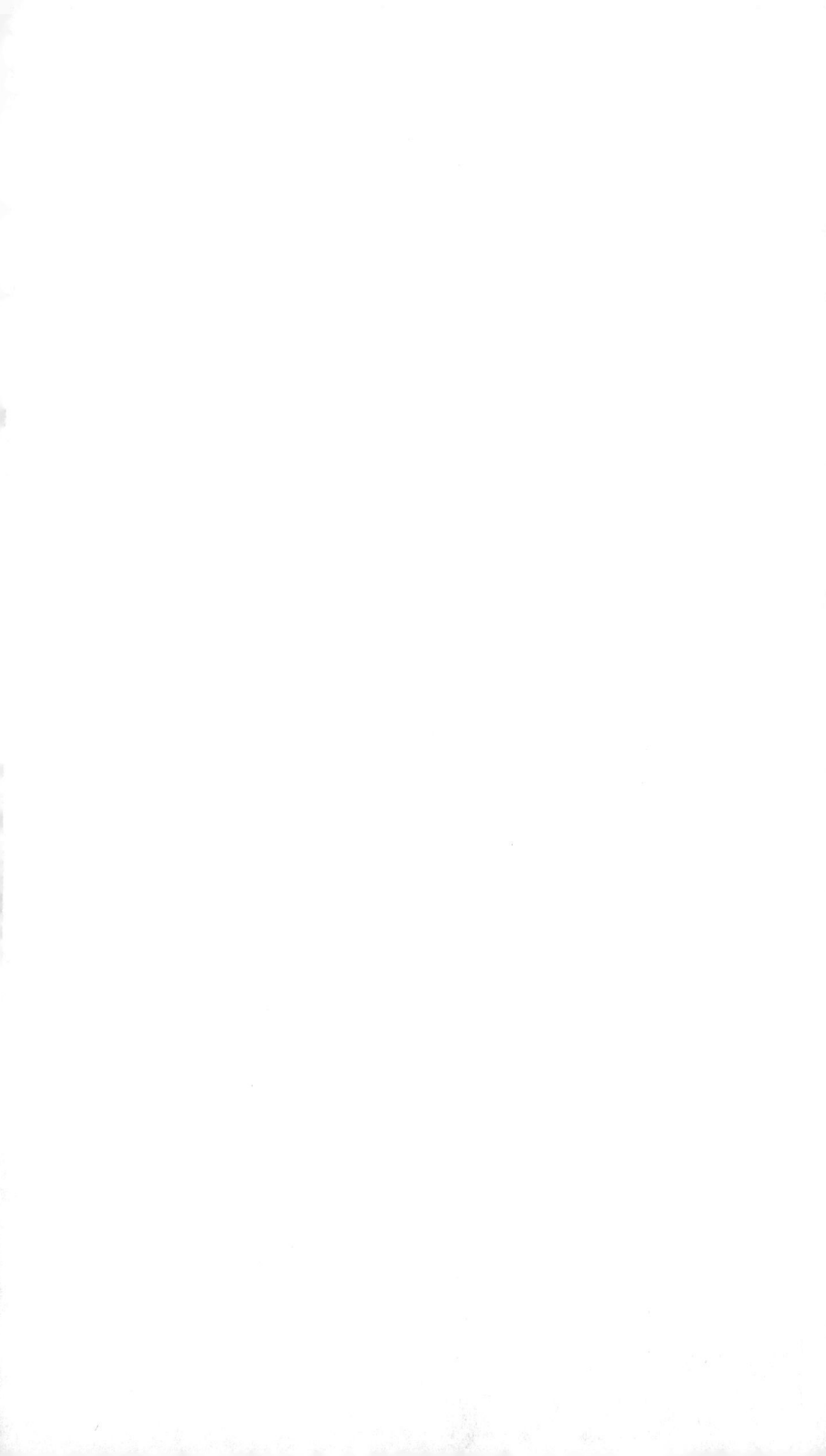

www.ingramcontent.com/pod-product-compliance
Lightning Source LLC
Chambersburg PA
CBHW060337050426
42449CB00011B/2782